Alvin Tomm

Dentistry: Dentistry and Implantology

Alvin Tomm

Dentistry: Dentistry and Implantology

Aesthetics and Rehabilitation

ScienciaScripts

Imprint
Any brand names and product names mentioned in this book are subject to trademark, brand or patent protection and are trademarks or registered trademarks of their respective holders. The use of brand names, product names, common names, trade names, product descriptions etc. even without a particular marking in this work is in no way to be construed to mean that such names may be regarded as unrestricted in respect of trademark and brand protection legislation and could thus be used by anyone.

Cover image: www.ingimage.com

This book is a translation from the original published under ISBN 978-613-9-62895-7.

Publisher:
Sciencia Scripts
is a trademark of
Dodo Books Indian Ocean Ltd. and OmniScriptum S.R.L publishing group

120 High Road, East Finchley, London, N2 9ED, United Kingdom
Str. Armeneasca 28/1, office 1, Chisinau MD-2012, Republic of Moldova, Europe
Printed at: see last page
ISBN: 978-620-7-75494-6

INDEX

INFLUENCE OF COLOR, SUBSTRATE AND TRANSLUCENCY ON THE FINAL RESULT OF CERAMIC VENEERS

The health sciences, especially dentistry, have come a long way in terms of technology, techniques and materials. In Restorative and Aesthetic Dentistry, adhesive techniques, knowledge about caries, etc. have shown a paradigm shift, **from "extension to prevention" to "minimally invasive preparations".**

Restorative dentistry is a blend of science and art. Success is determined on the basis of functional and aesthetic results (SIKRI, 2010). Aesthetics is currently sought after by increasingly demanding patients. The appearance of dental elements is a factor of great and growing importance for the majority of the population. The combination of colors not only improves aesthetics, but also makes restorations look natural and attractive (SIKRI, 2010). Thus, darkened teeth, due to a variety of causes, disturb an increasing number of patients who are looking for a beautiful smile.

Tooth darkening can have numerous causal factors, such as the absorption of pigments from the diet, poor dental formation, fluorosis, tetracycline staining, pulp hemorrhages, pigments from filling and restorative materials, deposition of secondary and tertiary dentin, reduction in enamel thickness, among others (WATTS; ADDY, 2001).

Darkened teeth can be treated in two ways. The treatment of choice is prophylaxis and tooth whitening (HILGERT, 2009). However, when darkened teeth show changes in shape, restorative treatments such as ceramic veneers are necessary. However, the interaction of the darkened substrate with the color of the restoration can affect the final color of the treatment.

Ideally, ceramic veneers should completely mask tooth discoloration with a minimum reduction in dental tissue of approximately 0.3 to 0.7mm. However, for severely discolored substrates, other devices should be used, such as the thickness of the restoration and the opacity of the material (CHU, 2009).

The choice of color during an aesthetic and rehabilitative treatment is a challenge for clinicians and specialists alike. Many components of the color choice process contribute to the difficulty of achieving a perfect match between the restoration and the rest of the dentition. Some of these factors stem from the subjective nature of human beings in relation to colors. In addition, fatigue, the aging and emotional state of the clinician, lighting conditions and metamerism add to the complexity of the task of choosing colors (CAL, GÜNERI, KOSE, 2006).

The aim of aesthetic and restorative dentistry is to create a beautiful smile, with teeth of pleasing proportions and an arrangement in harmony with the patient's gums, lips and face. Among the many difficulties in achieving this goal, color alteration of the substrate is one of them. The aim of this study was therefore to investigate *in vitro* the influence of ceramic shade, substrate and translucency on the final color of ceramic veneers.

LITERATURE REVIEW

CONSIDERATIONS ON CERAMIC VENEERS

Ceramic laminates offer a restorative solution that balances functional and aesthetic needs in the anterior dentition, and the clinician should always be able to make them (CLAVIJO, 2008).

Dental ceramics are widely used materials in dentistry. Chemical stability, high compressive strength, excellent and long-lasting aesthetics, and biocompatibility with the lowest plaque rates are some of the incomparable characteristics of ceramics (DELLA BONA, 2009).

Pincus, in 1947, was a clinician linked to the Beverly Hills art scene, and was much sought after by make-up artists to mask the aesthetic problems related to the teeth of some film stars. The author developed a technique that can be considered the forerunner of laminate veneers. Lost or aesthetically compromised teeth were temporarily covered with an acrylic or porcelain veneer, without any dental preparation and fixed with a powder, which limited the application to just a few hours (CLAVIJO, 2008).

The search for new restorative solutions in dentistry has driven the development and improvement of new restorative materials and techniques. In this new philosophy, one of the greatest concerns of the dental surgeon is to combine functionality and preservation of the dental structure with superior aesthetics (CLAVIJO, 2008).

In this way, the advancement of adhesion mechanisms in the various restorative materials contributes to an excellent aesthetic result. The use of adhesive systems allows for the preservation of healthy dental tissues, increasing patient awareness of the benefits of maintaining the structure of natural teeth and less invasive procedures. The restorative decision between veneers and crowns is extremely important in terms of **the "biological cost" of the** preparations required. Edelhoff and Sorensen (2002) simulated various types of preparation on artificial anterior teeth and, through thermogravimetric analysis, showed that the tooth reduction required for a veneer preparation is between 16.6 and 30.2% of the weight of the dental crown, while wear of between 62.8 and 72.1% is required to prepare a crown. One of the great assets that has boosted the success of veneers is their conservative nature compared to crowns. Veneers allow the palatal face to be preserved, which is extremely important for the distribution of occlusal forces and the consequent resistance of the dental element. Tissue preservation respects the principle of the possibility and ease of reintervention so that, in the event of future failure of the restoration (lifetime of the restoration), which is very likely in young patients, there are conditions to carry out a new treatment without, due to extensive dental destruction, the need to use more complex techniques or the loss of the dental element.

Gonzales et. al. (2011) reviewed the literature on laminate veneer restoration failures in journals listed on Pubmed from 1990 to 2010. These included longitudinal studies, reviews and in vitro research. To facilitate understanding, the study was divided and commented on in specific stages, where, according to the literature, the main failures of the laminate veneer technique are observed: case planning, selection of materials, types and techniques of preparation, treatment of tooth/restoration surfaces, cementation and longevity of the procedure. The first possible failure of this technique is the wrong selection of the case, as respect for its indications is an indispensable condition for successful treatment.

Comparative longitudinal studies lasting 5 to 10 years all show favorable results only for porcelain veneers, with an average success rate of 95 to 99%. However, there are several types of ceramic and it is important to know their characteristics so that there is less chance of error when choosing the material for each clinical situation. Thus, veneers are indicated for restorations of dental elements with: changes in color, shape, size, position, on vestibular faces with carious lesions or deficient restorations and for closing diastemas. Another indication would be the alteration and correction of occlusal relationships such as changing the guide and vertical dimension (GONZALES, 2011).

According to Vichi et. al. (2000) darkened substrates can negatively affect the esthetics of ceramic restorations. To this end, 1.0, 1.5 and 2.0 mm thick IPS-Empress discs were made and tested on simulated carbon fiber substrates, zirconia, an experimental substrate and an A3 colored composite substrate (Z100, 3M). The following aspects were evaluated: 1) the ceramic's ability to mask the substrate in relation to its thickness; 2) the effect of the color of the cement; 3) the influence of the thickness of the cement. When the ceramic thickness was 1.0mm, all the variables were visualized. For a thickness of 1.5mm, the differences in color were small and could only be identified with laboratory instruments. For the 2.0mm thickness, no differences were detected. In conclusion, the thickness of 2.0mm does not affect the final result of the restoration. When the thickness is reduced to 1.5mm, an analysis of the substrate is recommended in order to obtain the best result. When the thickness of the ceramic is 1.0mm, it is contraindicated to mask darkened substrates and the final result is affected.

When there is a need to mask dark backgrounds, one or more of the following options should be used: less translucent ceramics, greater thickness of restorative material, high quality cementing agents, etc.

opacity, low-translucency ceramic infrastructures covered with layered ceramics, among others (HIGERT, 2009).

There is an inversely proportional relationship between the thickness of a material and its degree of translucency. The thicker a translucent material, the greater its masking capacity, until a certain thickness is reached, called infinite optical thickness, in which the background no longer has any influence on the surface color, i.e. masking is complete. This is based on the Kubelka-Munk theory, which states that the infinite optical thickness of a given material varies according to its thickness and its diffusion and absorption rates for a given wavelength of the light spectrum. Thus, applying the basic idea of the Kubelka-Munk theory to the restoration of darkened teeth, it can be stated that: 1. a translucent dental restorative material can provide good masking, provided it is used in greater thickness. 2. reducing the degree of translucency of the restorative material helps to reduce the infinite optical thickness (HILGERT, 2009).

COLOR CONSIDERATIONS

Hue, Value and Chroma

Among the elements that make up the aesthetics of a smile, tooth color is of great importance (JARAD, 2008). Color is a psychophysical phenomenon, that is, it is the brain's response to a light stimulus captured by the eyes (AHMAD, 1999; AHMAD, 2000; PARAVINA; POWERS, 2004). The cones and rods of the human retina have photopigments which undergo a chemical transformation when they absorb certain wavelengths of the spectrum. The rods are greater in number, but are unable to provide information about colors. Colors are determined by cones, which can be of the S, M or L type (short-wave, medium-wave and long-wave), sensitive to short, medium and long waves respectively. The existence of three types of cones responsible for interpreting colors means that human color perception is three-dimensional (PARAVINA, POWERS, 2004). A person with normal vision can remember approximately 300 colors and is able to discriminate between 5 and 10 million different colors side by side (DELLA BONA, 2009).

Opaque objects receive light or the three primary colors (red, green and blue) in some proportion. Some of these objects reflect all the light they receive and others absorb almost all of it. Most **"opaque"** objects partially absorb and reflect the rest. The dominant wavelength reflected back to the eye is the color of the object. A white sheet of paper reflects almost all the light it receives. A black object absorbs most of the light. A perfectly black body is basically unaffected by a ray of light falling on it. A yellow object, when illuminated by the primary colors, absorbs blue and reflects green and red, which when mixed will appear as yellow (FONDRIEST, 2003).

Albert Munsell described color as a three-dimensional phenomenon. He described the three dimensions of color as hue, chroma and value. Hue is the quality that distinguishes one color family from another. Hue is specified as the dominant wavelength range in the visible spectrum that produces the perceived color, even though the exact wavelength of the perceived color may not be present. Hue is a physiological and psychological interpretation of a sum of wavelengths. In dental terms, hue is represented by the letters A, B, C or D on the VITA Color Scale. Value (brightness) is the amount of light returning from an object. Munsell described the value as a scale from white to black on a gray scale. Bright objects (high value) have a lower amount of gray while objects with a low value have a high amount of gray and appear dark. Some colors have a larger value range than others, maintaining their identity as they become darker. For example, blue remains recognizable as blue, even when an amount of grey is added. Yellow and orange, on the other hand, lose their hue identities when the value is lowered. The low value of a tooth's cervical is a difficult place to assess hue because of this. Chroma is the saturation, intensity or strength of the hue. Imagine putting red food coloring in a glass of water. Each time more dye is added, the intensity, saturation, chroma is increased. As more dye is added, the darker the mixture appears. When the chroma is increased, the value is decreased. Chroma and value are inversely related. On the VITA color scale, chroma is represented by numbers (FONDRIEST, 2003).

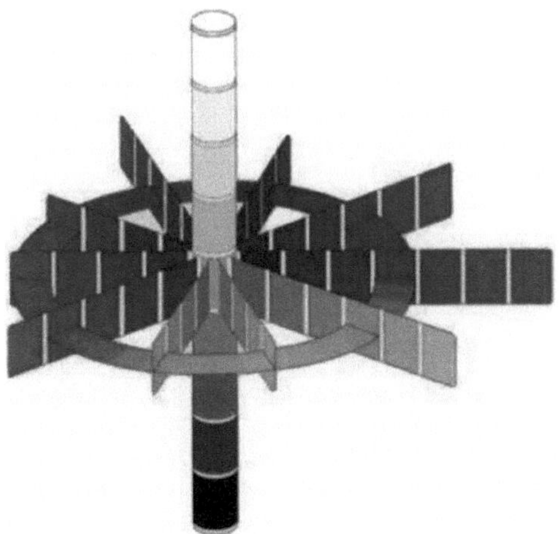

Figure 1: Representation of Munsell's color ordering system

The CIE (Commission Internationale de l'Eclairage) ordering system is the most widely used system for specifying colors. The observers, as well as the types of cones in the retina, are three: X, Y and Z. Just as certain wavelengths sensitize the S, M and L cones, the spectra captured by devices such as spectrophotometers are transformed into X, Y and Z tristimuli. Since the tristimuli represent the quantity of the additive primary colors (red, green, blue, or longwave, mediumwave and shortwave, respectively) it is possible, from the values of X, Y and Z, to numerically describe the color of an object for a specific illuminant (HILGERT, 2009).

To make the tristimulus system agree with Munsell's, the values of X, Y and Z were transformed, creating the CIELAB color ordering system (PARAVINA, POWERS, 2004).

In the CIELAB color space there is a luminosity scale, L*, (in which 0=absolute black and 100=absolute white), a scale on the green-red axis of opposites, a*, and a scale on the blue-yellow axis of opposites, b*. One of the most widespread uses of the CIELAB color space is for calculating the color difference between two samples (PARAVINA, R.; POWERS, J. 2004).

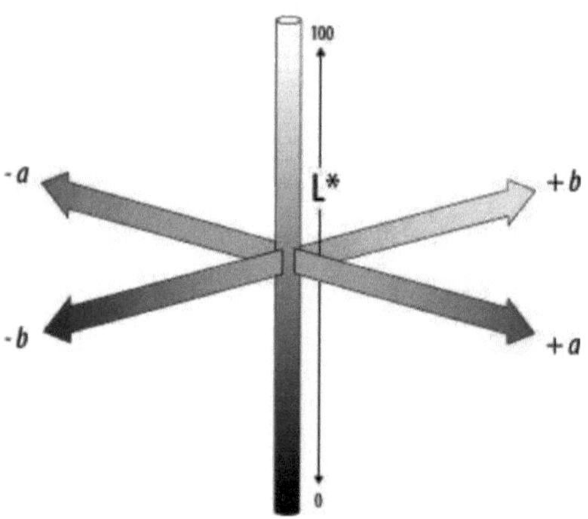

Figure 2: Color space representation of the CIELAB system

Translucency

In ceramic restorations, the attempt to imitate the appearance of the natural tooth consists of the sum of all the color dimensions (hue, chroma and value). However, in addition to these dimensions, there are other variables that also influence the final color, including translucency. Translucency can be defined as the gradient between transparent and opaque (FONDRIEST, 2003).

The optical behavior of teeth is directly related to the individual characteristics of the tissues that form them: enamel and dentin. Human teeth are characterized by different degrees of translucency, which can be defined as the gradient between transparent and opaque. Generally, increasing the translucency of a restoration reduces its value, as it returns less light to the eye. With increased translucency, light is able to pass from the surface and spread within the restoration (SIKRI, V.K, 2010). According to Raptis et. al. (2006), enamel is considered to be translucent

It can transmit over 70% of the incident light through a 1mm thick section, and approximately 97% of the mass of human enamel is made up of organized hydroxyapatite crystals. Dentin, however, has around 70% of these crystals arranged in a tubular shape, which is why dentin is less translucent than enamel and can transmit 30% of the light incident on a 1mm thick specimen (PINTO, 2009). Similarly to what happens in dental tissues and other materials, a beam of light is attenuated when it passes through a ceramic solid, as light interacts with the material's intrinsic absorption and scattering by optical heterogeneities. The main optical heterogeneities are surfaces, secondary phases (including pores) and, in polycrystalline ceramics, grain contours (PINTO, 2009).

Spectrophotometer

Traditionally, shade selection is done by visual comparison of an object (the tooth) with shade scales (CAL, GÜNERI, KOSE, 2006). Another way of obtaining the color of teeth and restorations is by the spectrophotometric method.

The same color can be perceived differently by different observers. It is therefore possible for a color identification instrument to remove subjectivity in color perception. One of the **instruments used for this purpose is an "intraoral spectrophotometer"** (EasyShade®, Vita) with specifications for identifying two commercial color scales: Vita-3D-Master (Vita) and Vitapan Classical (Vita). This combination of color scales, instrumental development and calibration capacity present in these devices provides an orderly and integrated testing system (DELLA BONA, 2009).

Spectrophotometers measure and record the amount of light reflected or transmitted by an object, and the data must be transformed into a useful format such as spectral curves (CHU; DEVIGUS; MIELESZKO, 2004).

The word spectrophotometry refers to a method of analysis based on measurements of the absorption of electromagnetic radiation. This technique is restricted to a small wavelength region of electromagnetic radiation, which corresponds to visible or ultraviolet light: it is the range between approximately 200 and 700nm (1 nanometer = 10-9m, **700nm = 0.7µm) (HIRATA, 2008).**

A typical spectrophotometer consists of a light source, a monochromator and a detector. The light source is usually a deuterium or xenon lamp, which emits electromagnetic radiation in the UV region of the spectrum. A second light source, usually a tungsten lamp, is used for wavelengths in the visible region of the spectrum. The monochromator is a diffraction network; its function is to separate the light beam into its constituent wavelengths. A system of slits focuses the desired wavelength on the sample. The radiation passes through the sample and reaches the detector, which registers the intensity of the transmitted light. The sample holder must be made of material that is transparent in the visible range to the electromagnetic radiation used in the experiment. In the case of spectroscopy in the visible range, sample cells (or cuvettes, square tubes) made of glass or plastic are used. For measurements in the ultraviolet region, quartz cuvettes are used, a material that does not absorb radiation in the ultraviolet range (HIRATA, 2008).

Dozic et. al. (2007) reported that EasyShade was the most reliable instrument *in in-vivo* and *in-vivo* studies. However, the relationship between visual observation and instrumental identification for taking color needs further study. There is little research comparing visual observation with instrumental identification.

Dark substrate

A basic understanding of the elements of tooth color is important for many aspects of restorative dentistry. Teeth are typically composed of numerous colors and the gradation of these occurs on a tooth from the gingival margin towards the incisal edge (WATTS, A.; ADDY, M. 2001).

The coronal portion of the tooth is made up of enamel, dentin and pulp. Any change in these structures is likely to cause a change in the external appearance of the tooth. The color of the tooth is dependent on the quality of the reflected light and is also, as a consequence, dependent on the incident light (WATTS, A.; ADDY, M. 2001).

Historically, tooth discoloration has been classified according to the location of the darkening, which can be intrinsic or extrinsic. Another category of discoloration that can be considered is internalized staining (ADDY M, MORAN J.1995).

Intrinsic discoloration occurs after a structural change or due to a reduction in the thickness of dental tissues. A large number of metabolic and systemic diseases can affect tooth development and cause discoloration as a result. Examples include amelogenesis imperfecta, dentinogenesis imperfecta, fluorosis, tetracycline stain, enamel hypoplasia, among others (WATTS, A.; ADDY, M. 2001).

Extrinsic discoloration occurs on the external surface of the tooth and is found on the surface or in the acquired film, and can be of metallic or non-metallic origin (WATTS, A.; ADDY, M. 2001).

Internalized stains are the incorporation of extrinsic stains into the tooth structure after development. This occurs due to defects in the enamel and also due to the exposure of dentin. The routes by which pigments can become internalized are developmental defects or acquired defects such as tooth wear, gingival recession, decay and restorative materials (WATTS, A.; ADDY, M. 2001).

Based on the existing literature, it can be seen that the masking capacity has not yet been systematically studied using the main ceramic materials currently available and varying the thickness within clinically relevant limits (PINTO, 2009). Therefore, the aim of this study is to investigate *in vitro* the influence of substrate color, thickness and ceramic translucency on the final color of ceramic veneers.

OBJECTIVES

-       To investigate *in vitro* the influence of ceramic color, substrate and translucency on the final color of ceramic veneers.

-       To evaluate, *in vitro,* using a spectrophotometer, the final result of ceramic veneers with different colors and translucency on a darkened substrate.

METHODOLOGY

DELINEATION

Experimental study *in vitro,* carried out at the CEOM/Imed Postgraduate Unit.

SAMPLE

Two stock teeth (P-Oclusal, Brazil), upper central incisors (21), one in color A3 and the other with a darkened substrate in color C4, were used in a plastic mannequin (P-Oclusal, Brazil), prepared for slides in a standardized way.

PROCEDURES

The preparation of the simulated substrates began with the preparation of ceramic veneers for plastic teeth from the P-Oclusal NS1 mannequin for element 21 with 1.0mm of wear.

For this *in vitro* study, four e.max CAD HT (*High Translucency*) and LT (*Low Translucency*) *veneers were* used, two in shade A2 and the other two in shade A3, for tooth 21. The *try-in* paste *Variolink® Veneer* (Ivoclar Vivadent) in shade 0 was used to cement the *veneers.* The variation of the groups is described in the images below:

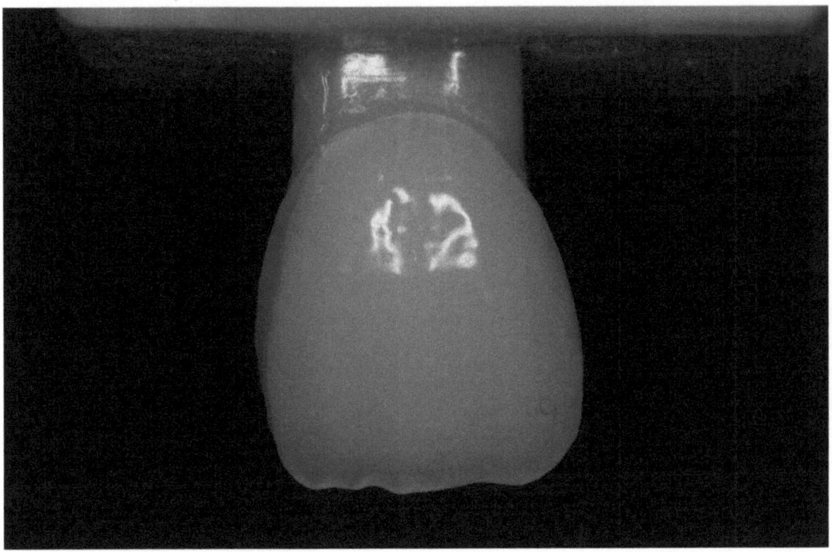

Figure 3: Tooth-Face A2 HT (control)

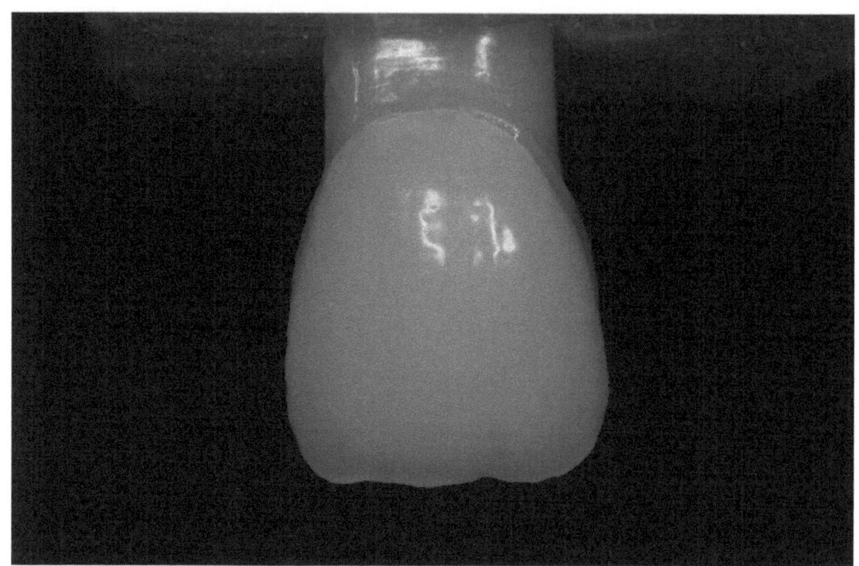

Figure 4: Tooth-Face A2 LT

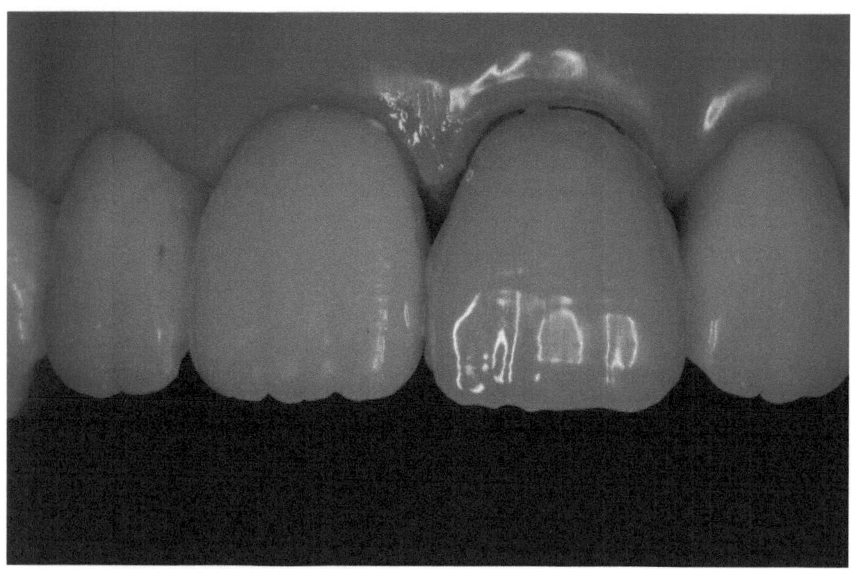

Figure 5: Tooth-Face A2 HT - E

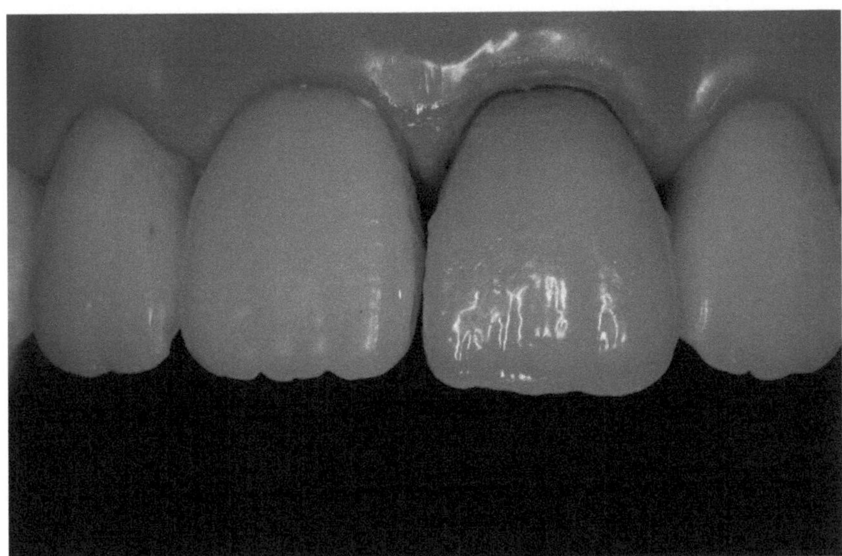

Figure 6: Tooth-Face A2 LT - E

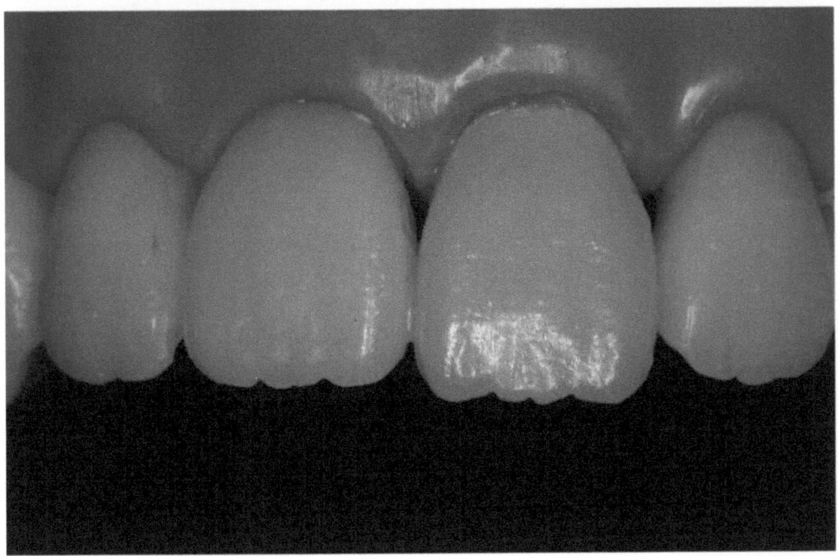

Figure 7: Tooth-Face A3 HT (control)

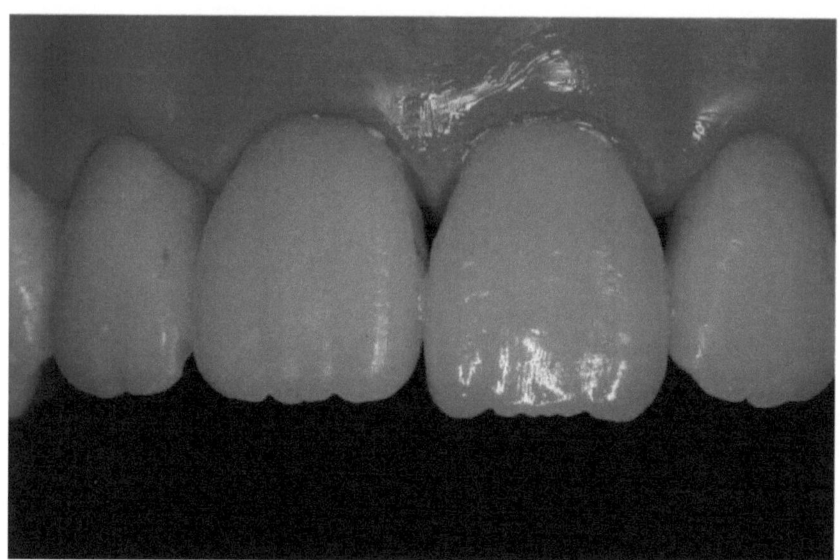

Figure 8: Tooth-Face A3 LT

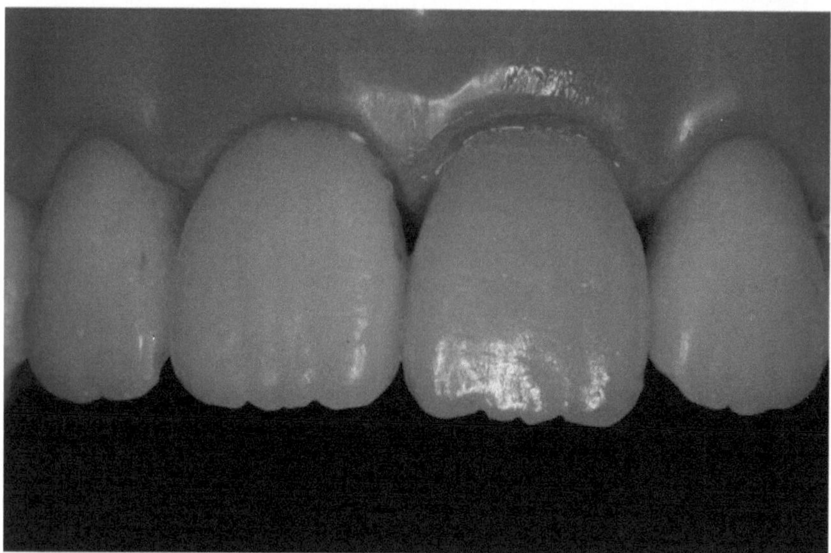

Figure 9: Tooth-Face A3 HT - E

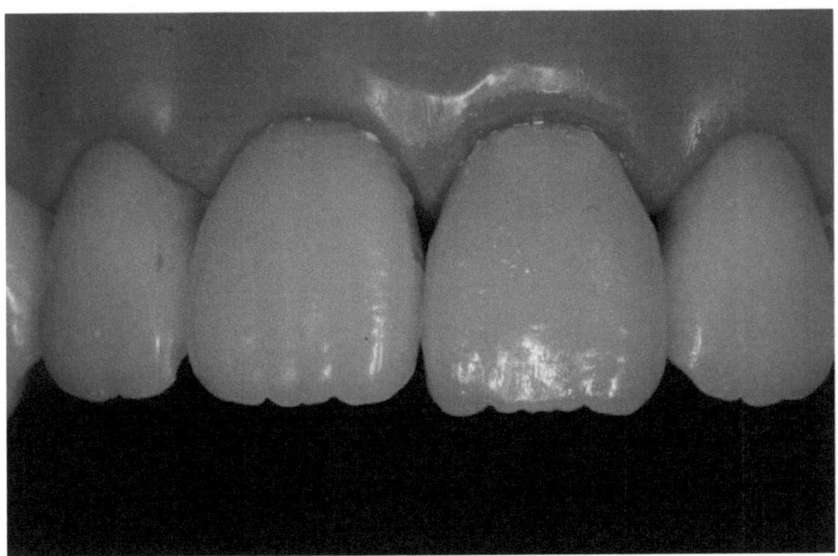

Figure 10: Tooth-Face A3 LT - E

Taking into account the variation in veneer color, translucency and substrate, the groups were divided as follows:

- Group 1 = A2 HT (control)

- Group 2 = A2LT

- Group 3 = A2HT - E

- Group 4 = A2LT - E

- Group 5 = A3HT (control)

- Group 6 = A3LT

- Group 7 = A3HT - E

- Group 8 = A3LT - E

The try-in paste *Variolink® Veneer* (Ivoclar Vivadent) was used to fix the *veneers to* the tooth. The veneer for group 1 was positioned first. After removing the excess with a *microbrush* and dental floss, the tooth-veneer set was photographed. This procedure was also carried out on the remaining groups.

Spectrophotometric evaluation

After the groups had been prepared, they were evaluated spectrophotometrically. The device used was the VITA EasyShade (VITA) (ES). To obtain the values for each group, two shots were taken with the ES, one with a normal substrate and the other with a darkened substrate. The color difference, represented by the expression Δ**E,** is calculated using the formula:

$$\Delta E = (\Delta L^{*2} + \Delta a^{*2} + \Delta b^{*2})_{1/2}$$

Where Δ**L*= difference between the brightness of the samples;** a*= difference on the a* scale (green-red) **between the samples; and** b*= difference on the b* scale (blue-yellow) between the samples. **The** Δ**E value** adopted for this study was 3.3.

The use of the CIELAB color difference calculation is widespread in dentistry, both in vitro and in vivo. The vast majority of studies that have tried to simulate the effect of restorative materials on darkened backgrounds, however, have used flat, polished disk-shaped specimens (HILGERT, 2009). In the present study, the methodology used is the spectrophotometric evaluation of the groups, correlating them with clinical situations.

Each veneer-substrate group was evaluated three times. The L*, a* and b* coordinates were taken from the middle third of the buccal face of the specimens. The average of the three shots is the color of the specimen. The data obtained was stored and calculated in an electronic spreadsheet (Excel 2010, Microsoft).

RESULTS

Spectrophotometric color analysis

The averages of the data obtained from the three evaluations of the study groups using the spectrophotometer are shown in Table 1. The raw data obtained from the spectrophotometer can be found in Appendix A.

Average		L*		a*		b*
A2 HT (control)		79,16667		-1		10,93333
A2 LT		82		-1,46667		17,13333
A3 HT (control)		78,4		-0,2		15,43333
A3 LT		78,93333		0,233333		20,7
A2 HT - E		73,86667		0,2		10,73333
A2 LT - E		76,36667		-0,2		16,4
A3 HT - E		77,5		-0,23333		13,5
A3 LT - E		77,4		0,433333		18,93333

Table 1: Study group averages

Each specimen had its L*a*b* coordinates (average of three spectrophotometric measurements) compared with the average values of the reference restoration using the following formulas, resulting in differences in each of the coordinates (L*, a* and b*):

(1) **ΔL*= L*Measured** - L*Restoration Reference

(2) **Δa*= a*Measured** - a*Restoration Reference

(3) **Δb*= b*Measured** - b*Restoration Reference

Based on these values, the color difference (E) between each specimen and the reference restoration was calculated using the formula:

$$\Delta E = (\Delta L^{*2} + \Delta a^{*2} + \Delta b^{*2})_{1/2}$$

Table 2 shows the average **ΔL*, a*, b* and E** values for each combination of Substrate, Translucency and Ceramic Color.

Groups	ΔL*		Δa*	Δb*	ΔE
A2 HT (control)	79,16		-1	10,93	0
A2 LT	2,84		-0,46	6,2	4,28
A3 HT (control)	78,4		-0,2	15,43	0
A3 LT	0,53		0,43	5,27	2,97
A2 HT - E	-5,3		1,2	-0,2	4,13
A2 LT - E	-2,8		0,8	5,47	4,1
A3 HT - E	-1,66		0,77	2,57	1,33
A3 LT - E	-1,76		1,43	8	2,22

Table 2: **Average ΔL*,** a*, b* **and E values for each** Substrate **combination,**

Translucency and color of ceramics.

DISCUSSION

Advances in the understanding of adhesion mechanisms have boosted the success of veneers. The concept of conditioned ceramics was introduced in 1982 by Simonsen and Calamia. These authors reported that the bond strength between tooth and restoration was sufficient for the retention of ceramic veneers (CALAMIA 1985). Today, the techniques used to fix veneers are well-established. Ideally, the aim is to preserve the enamel for a long-lasting adhesive bond. In this sense, Peumans et. al. (2004) in a study of the clinical evaluation of veneers with five to ten years of cementation. The results showed that, after ten years, no veneers had been lost. The percentage of restorations **that were considered "clinically acceptable" was 92% after five years and 64% after ten years. Only 4% were considered "clinically unacceptable" after 10 years. This study**

corroborates the results of other authors (GRANELL-RUIZ, M et.al. 2010; GUESS, STAPPERT, 2007). These data suggest that veneers are a conservative treatment, in which the palatal side of the tooth is preserved, increasing longevity and also making intervention possible, should the need arise.

Another relevant factor for veneers is cementation. The color of a ceramic restoration is the result of the interaction between the substrate and the veneer (LEE, Y. et. al. 2007). Due to the different thicknesses that veneers can be made in, the cementing agent also has a major influence on the final color result. The smaller the thickness, the greater the prevalence of the substrate's color. When the substrate has a color change, the cementing agent must prevent this unpleasant factor. In this study, we opted not to include cementation as a variable, so we used a medium-value *try-in* gel.

Difficulties in choosing a shade are prevalent in restorative dentistry. For treatment to be fully successful, color is an important factor. A person with normal vision is able to distinguish approximately 300 different colors (DELLA BONA, 2009). The impression of color with the naked eye is very subjective, not measurable and therefore perceived and felt differently by each individual (HUGO, WITZEL,

KLAIBER, 2005). This subjectivity imposed on obtaining the correct treatment color has led to the creation of devices that remove the human factor from the choice. Spectrophotometers are devices that eliminate subjectivity from the process, making it possible to obtain the correct shade. Dozic et. al. (2007) tested five commercial spectrophotometers under *in vitro* and *in vivo* conditions. In conclusion, the EasyShade (VITA) and Ikam (DCM) devices gave the most reliable results. The other devices had better results in the *in vitro* tests. The EasyShade spectrophotometer (VITA) was the same one used in this study. However, it is suggested that future research correlate visual evaluation with spectrophotometric evaluation, since the same human factor that has difficulty choosing a shade can discern whether the restoration is an acceptable shade, both for the professional and the patient.

Darkened substrates are a challenge for restorations with ceramic veneers. Due to the passage of light through the ceramic, the color of the remnant affects the final result of the treatment. The major challenge in achieving an excellent esthetic result is to mask the dark background without making the restoration opaque. According to the Kubella-Munk theory, the thicker a translucent material, the greater its masking capacity, until **"infinite optical thickness" is reached, in which the background no longer has any** influence on the color of the surface (HILGERT, 2009). As enamel is highly translucent, veneers should behave in the same way. An excessively opaque material, in addition to influencing cementation, due to a more invasive preparation in which enamel is removed and dentin is exposed, has an optical behavior that is inverse to that of the natural tooth, affecting aesthetics. The success of treatment with veneers on darkened substrates seems to lie in the balance between the depth of preparation and the opacity of the restorative materials (HILGERT, 2009). Figure 11 summarizes the main problems pointed out in the literature when treating darkened teeth with ceramic veneers. These problems are related to the interrelationship between ceramic thickness, material translucency and substrate color in the final aesthetic result of restorations.

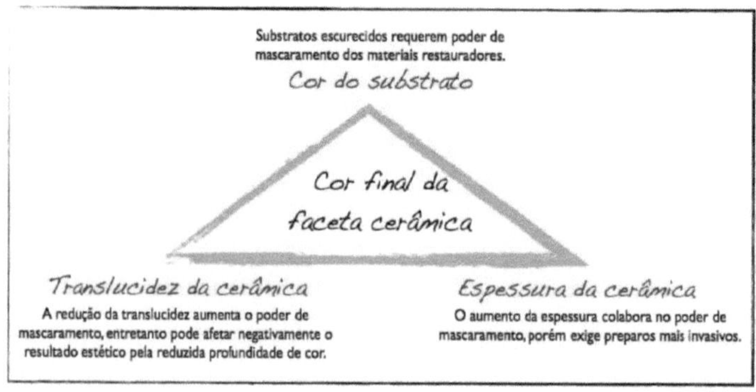

Figure 11: Representation of the relationship between substrate color, thickness and ceramic translucency on the final color of laminate veneers (HILGERT et al. 2009).

The use of the CIELAB color space and the color measurements by the **ΔE calculation** formula used are considered standards within dentistry and have a proven good relationship with visual observations (PARAVINA, R.D.; POWERS, J.M, 2004). The ΔE reference value used in this study was 3.3. This value is similar to that proposed by other authors (HILGERT, 2009; PINTO, 2009).

In this study, the difference in the color of the specimens was more prevalent in the A2-colored veneers. In these restorations, the substrate and translucency had an effect on the final color. For A3 veneers, the substrate had no influence on the final color, regardless of translucency. The **A2 restorations had a** ΔE **greater than 3.3, even for normal substrates. Studies indicate that a** ΔE **of up to 6.8 was clinically acceptable to clinical** evaluators (JOHNSTON; KAO, 1989). For the A2 shade groups, the values were 4.23 (LT), 4.13 (HT - E) and 4.10 (LT - E). Based on the results obtained by spectrophotometric analysis, it is believed that these **restorations with a** higher ΔE were due to lower chroma saturation. The low translucency veneer leaves the restoration with a higher value. The A3 color veneers showed no difference in ΔE values. The higher chroma saturation of the A3 veneers seems to have interfered with the lack of a visible color difference, i.e. greater than 3.3.

Ceramic veneers have proven their worth over the years, as they are currently a fashionable form of treatment. The longevity and aesthetics that this treatment offers patients are undeniable. However, as ceramics are generally highly translucent and have a thickness of around 0.7 to 1.0mm, the substrate has a major influence on the final result of the restorative treatment. A darkened substrate negatively affects the color of the ceramic surface. More invasive preparations can mitigate this factor, however this increase in the thickness of the ceramic can lead to greater opacity of the material.

CONCLUSION

In view of the above, we conclude that:

-       The color of the veneer influences the final color of the restoration.

-       A2-colored veneers on a darkened substrate showed a $\Delta E > 3.3$ and the color difference was perceptible to the human eye.

-       For A2 coloured veneers, the darkened substrate and translucency interfere with the final result.

-       For A3 coloured veneers, regardless of translucency, the darkened substrate does not interfere with the final result.

-       Further studies linking spectrophotometric evaluations with visual evaluations are suggested.

REFERENCES

ADDY M, MORAN J. Mechanisms of stain formation on teeth, in particular associated with metal ions and antiseptics. *Advances in Dental Research.* Washington. v.9, p. 450-456,1995.

AHMAD, I. Three-Dimensional Shade Analysis: Perspectives of Color Part I. *Practical Periodontics and Aesthetic Dentistry*, New York, v.11, n.7, p.789-96, Sep.1999.

AHMAD, I. Three-Dimensional Shade Analysis: Perspectives of Color Part II. *Practical Periodontics and Aesthetic Dentistry*, New York, v.12, n.6, p.557-64, 2000.

BUONOCORE, M.G. A simple method of increasing the adhesion of acrylic filling materials to enamel surfaces. *Journal of dental research.* Washington, v.34, p.849-53, 1955.

CAL, E, GÜNERI, P, KOSE, T. Comparison of digital and spectrophotometric measurements of color shade guides. *Journal of Oral Rehabilitation.* Oxford, v. 33, p. 221-228.

CALAMIA, J. R. Etched porcelain veneers: the current state of the art. *Quintessence int.* v. 16, n. 1, p. 5-12, 1985.

CHU, F.C. Clinical considerations in managing severe tooth discoloration with porcelain veneer. *JADA*, Chicago, v.140, p.442-446, 2009.

CHU, J. DEVIGUS, A., MIELESZKO, A. *The physics of color in Fundamentals of color: Shade Matching and communication in esthetic dentistry.* Chicago: Ed. Quinteessence: 2004.

CLAVIJO, V. et. al. Ceramic laminates. *International Journal of Brazilian Dentistry*, Florianópolis, v.4, n.2, p. 164-173, apr./jun. 2008

DOZIC, A, et. al. **Performance of five commercially available toothcolormeasuring** devices. *Journal of Prosthodontics,* Philadelphia, n.16, p.**93-100**, 2007.

DELLA BONA, et. al. Visual and instrumental agreement in dental shade selection: Three distinct observer populations and shade matching protocols. *Dental material,* Washington, n. 25, p. **276-281**, 2009.

DELLA BONA, A. *Adhesion to ceramics:* scientific evidence for clinical use. Sao Paulo: Artes Médicas; 2009.

EDELHOFF, D.; SORENSEN, J.A. Tooth structure removal associated with various preparation designs for anterior teeth. *Journal of prosthetic dentistry*, St. Louis, v.87, p.503-9, 2002.

FONDRIEST, J. Shade Matching in Restorative Dentistry: The Science & Strategies. *Int J Periodontics Restorative Dent.* Chicago. v. 23, n. 5, p. 467-479. 2003.

GUESS, P.C.; STAPPERT, C.F. Midterm results of a 5-year prospective clinical investigation of extended ceramic veneers. *Dent Mater*, Washigton. v.24, p.804813, 2007.

GONZALEZ, M.R, et. al. Failures in restorations with laminated veneers: a 20-year literature review. *Rev. bras. odontol.*, Rio de Janeiro, v. 68, n. 2, p. 238-43, Jul./Dec. 2011.

GRANELL-RUIZ, M et.al. A clinical longitudinal study 323 porcelain laminate veneers. Period of study from 3 to 11 years. Med Oral Patol Oral Cir Bucal. Valencia. v. 3, n 1, p. 531-537. 2010.

HIRATA, R. *Evaluation of reflectance, direct transmittance and fluorescence of composite resins.* 2008. 115 f. Thesis (Doctorate in Dentistry) School of Dentistry, Rio de Janeiro State University, Rio de Janeiro, 2008.

HUGO, B., WITZEL, T., KLAIBER, B. Comparison of in vivo visual and computer-aided tooth shade determination. *Clin Oral Invest.* v. 9, p. **244-250**, 2005.

HILGERT, L. A. *Influence of Substrate Color, Thickness and Translucency of the Ceramic on the Final Color of Laminated Veneers Produced with the CEREC InLab System.* Florianópolis: UFSC, 2009. Thesis (Doctorate), Federal University of Santa Catarina-SC, Florianópolis, 2009.

HILGERT, L.A. et al. Influence of stump shade, ceramic thickness and translucency on the color of veneers. Dent Mater, Washington. v.25. p.9 , 2009.

JARAD, F.D. et. al. The Effect of Bleaching, Varying the Shade or Thickness of Composite Veneers on Final Color: an in vitro study. *Journal of Dentistry*, San Antonio, v.36, n.7, p.v554-559, Jul. 2008.

LEE, Y., CHA, H., AHN, J. Layered color of all-ceramic core and veneer ceramics. *J Prosthet Dent*, St. Louis. v. 97, p. 279-86, 2007.

PARAVINA, R. D.; POWERS, J.M. Esthetic Color Training in Dentistry. *Elsevier Mosby,* St. Louis. p. 245. 2004.

Peumans M, De Munck J, Fieuws S, Lambrechts P, Vanherle G, Van Meerbeek B. A prospective ten-year clinical trial of porcelain veneers. J Adhes Dent. 2004;6:65-76.

PINTO, M. M. *Optical properties and microstructure of ceramic dental restoration materials (thesis)*. Sao Paulo: University of Sao Paulo, Faculty of Dentistry, 2009.

RAPTIS, N.V., MICHALAKIS, K.X., HIRAYAMA, H. Optical behavior of current ceramic systems. *In J Per Rest. Dent.* Chicago, v. 1, n. 26, p. 31-41, 2006.

SIKRI, V.K. Color: Implications in dentistry. J Conserv Dent, Mumbai. n.13 p.249-55, 2010

VICHI, A., FERRARI, M., DAVIDSON C.L., In fluence of ceramic and cement thickness on the masking of various types of opaque posts. *Journal of prosthetic dentistry*, St. Louis, v. 83, n. 4, p. 412-417.

WATTS, A.; ADDY, M. Tooth discolouration and staining: a review of the literature. *British dental journal.* London. v.190, p.309-16, 2001.

APPENDIX

Appendix A

Raw data obtained from the spectrophotometer

Groups (take 1)	L*	a*	b*
A2 HT (control)	79,1	-1	10,9
A2 LT	82.7	-1,5	17,2
A3 HT (control)	78.5	-0,1	15,7
A3 LT	79.1	0,1	20,5
A2 HT - E	74.0	0.2	10,8
A2 LT - E	76.4	-0,2	16,4
A3 HT - E	78.7	-0,3	13,8
A3 LT - E	78.4	0,3	18,7
Groups (take 2)	L*	a*	b*
A2 HT (control)	79,2	-1	10,9
A2 LT	81.6	-1,4	17,2
A3 HT (control)	78.2	-0,3	15,2
A3 LT	78.7	0,2	20,7
A2 HT - E	73.6	0,3	10,9
A2 LT - E	76.0	-0,2	16,3
A3 HT - E	76.7	-0,3	13,4
A3 LT - E	76.7	0,5	19
Groups (take 3)	L*	a*	b*
A2 HT (control)	79,2	-1	11
A2 LT	81,7	-1,5	17
A3 HT (control)	78,5	-0,2	15,4
A3 LT	79	0,4	20,9
A2 HT - E	74	0,1	10,5
A2 LT - E	76,7	-0,2	16,5
A3 HT - E	77,1	-0,1	13,3
A3 LT - E	77,1	0,5	19,1

Appendix B

Color difference

Groups	First color			Second color			Differences			
	L	a	b	L	a	b	ΔL	Δa	Δb	ΔE00
A2 HT	79,16	-1,00	10,93	79,16	-1,00	10,93	0,00	0,00	0,00	0
A2 LT	82,00	-1,46	17,13	79,16	-1,00	10,93	2,84	0,46	6,20	4,28
A2HT - E	73,86	0,20	10,73	79,16	-1,00	10,93	5,30	1,20	0,20	4,13
A2 LT - E	76,36	-0,20	16,40	79,16	-1,00	10,93	2,80	0,80	5,47	4,10

A3 HT	78,40	-0,20	15,43	78,40		-0,20	15,43	0,00		0,00	0,00	0
A3 LT	78,93	0,23	20,70	78,40		-0,20	15,43	0,53		0,43	5,27	2,97
A3 HT - E	77,50	-0,23	13,50	78,40		-0,20	15,43	0,90		0,03	1,93	1,33
A3 LT - E	77,40	0,43	18,93	78,40		-0,20	15,43	1,00		0,63	3,50	2,22

GUIDED OSSEOUS REGENERATION IN THE AESTHETIC REGION - LITERATURE REVIEW

As a health science, dentistry has made great progress, both in terms of techniques and materials. Adhesive systems, resin composites that mimic dental tissues, ceramics that are highly resistant and aesthetically pleasing, among others, are some of the recent advances. In this way, implant dentistry has evolved rapidly in recent decades, with high predictability and success rates (WENNERBERG; ALBREKTSSON, 2011).

The loss of a single tooth for various reasons causes embarrassment and social discomfort (SHARMA et al., 2011). It is known that the lack of one or more teeth is related to not only aesthetic but also functional problems that trigger chewing and phonetic difficulties (AMOROSO et al., 2012).

Bone defects in the alveolar ridge, due to atrophy, periodontal disease and trauma sequelae, can result in insufficient bone volume, vertically and transversely, which can make implant placement impossible or incorrect from an aesthetic point of view (ALOY-PRÓSPER et al., 2015).

A deficiency of bone tissue in the buccal-lingual direction can make implant installation unfeasible, so various techniques have been proposed to promote an increase in bone tissue, such as autogenous grafts, alveolar distraction, among others, but with various disadvantages. Thus, Guided Bone Regeneration is an alternative in these cases, especially in regions involving the anterior maxilla.

Guided Bone Regeneration (GBR) is a procedure for reconstructing the alveolar ridge using membranes. This procedure is indicated when there is not enough bone tissue to place implants or in cases where aesthetics are required. GBR can be performed prior to implant placement, when there is insufficient bone tissue for initial implant stability and no predictable results, or simultaneously with implant placement. GBR is based on the principles of Guided Tissue Regeneration (GTR). GTR was first described by Nyman et al. in the early 1980s. This concept is based on the principle that specific cells contribute to the formation of specific tissues. Melcher described the concept of selective cell repopulation of defects to improve healing. With the exception of cells of epithelial and connective tissue origin, a periodontal wound, in 6-8 weeks, allows slow-growing tissues (osteoblasts, cementoblasts and periodontal ligament cells) to occupy the spaces adjacent to the teeth. GBR uses the same principles of excluding specific tissues, but not associated with the tooth. Thus, the term adopted for the technique was "Guided Bone

Regeneration" (FARZAD; MOHAMMADI, 2012).

Implant therapy is now widely regarded as a reliable treatment option for replacing lost teeth, both functionally and aesthetically. The original treatment protocols from the 1970s and 1980s required fully healed alveolar ridges before installing implants. In the 1990s, these protocols were modified to include implant placement in post-extraction alveoli or partially healed ridge predominantly for implants in the esthetic zone (CHEN; BUSER, 2014).

According to Chen and Buser (2014), the integrity of the buccal bone level can be an important factor in long-term esthetic stability. Also according to the authors, more research is needed to establish which are the most suitable materials for reconstructing the buccal bone and also the long-term stability of the gingival margin and the presence or absence of buccal bone and the position of the bone crest.

The aim of this study is therefore to investigate the predictability of guided bone regeneration in aesthetic areas, the stability of the treatment over time and also the comparison between different materials by means of a literature review of journals indexed in English and Portuguese databases from 2000 to 2015.

LITERATURE REVIEW

GUIDED BONE REGENERATION: WHAT IS IT?

Guided bone regeneration is based on the creation of a secreted space for the invasion of blood vessels and osteoprogenitor cells, protecting bone repair against the growth of non-osteogenic tissues that have a faster migration rate than osteogenic cells. It is a technique in which physical means, such as a membrane, are used to prevent other tissues, mainly connective tissue, from interfering with osteogenesis (DINATO et al., 2007).

Bone is a relatively slow-growing tissue, and both fibroblasts and epithelial cells have the opportunity to occupy the available space more efficiently and build up soft connective tissue much faster than bone is able to grow. Thus, the biological mechanism of GBR is the exclusion of undesirable cells in the space filled by the coagulum under the membrane (BUSER, 2010).

MEMBERS

The principle of physically excluding an anatomical site in order to improve the repair of a certain type of tissue and direct its regeneration, with some type of mechanical barrier, has been used in reconstructive surgery. In the case of bone reconstructive surgery, a barrier is used to prevent the invagination of soft connective tissue into the bone defect (BUSER, 2010).

The basic characteristics of membranes are: biocompatibility, cell occlusion, tissue integration, space formation and maintenance, clinical management in surgery and limited susceptibility to complications (MCALLISTER; HAGHIGTH, 2007).

Due to the risk of premature exposure and the need for a second surgery to remove the non-resorbable membranes, clinicians and researchers have advocated the use of resorbable membranes in GBR procedures (BUSER, 2010).

BONE GRAFTS AND SUBSTITUTE MATERIALS

Bone-filling materials serve several purposes in GBR, such as: they support the membrane, preventing it from collapsing; they act as a framework for bone invagination from the recipient bed; they stimulate bone invagination from the recipient bed; they provide a mechanical barrier against the pressure of the overlying soft tissue; they protect the increased volume from being resorbed (BUSER, 2010).

The classification of bone augmentation materials can be found in Table 1.

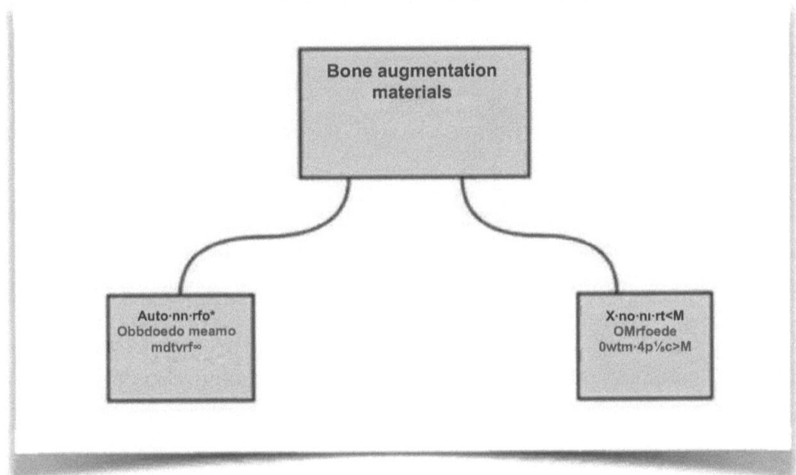

Source: Buser (2010 - adapted)

Autogenous bone

Autogenous bone is made up of around 30% and 70% organic and inorganic compounds, respectively. Of the organic compounds, 90% to 95% are collagen (type I) and the remainder is represented by non-collagenous proteins such as osteocalcin, calcitonin and sialoproteins. The inorganic component is made up predominantly of crystalline hydroxyapatite (HA) (BUSER, 2010).

In order to provide the best results, the graft should preferably be osteogenic, osteoinductive and osteoconductive (DELIBERADOR et al., 2006; FURLANETO et al., 2007). Osteogenesis occurs when viable osteoblasts form part of the graft and, with an adequate blood supply at the grafted site, form ossification centers. Osteoinduction involves new bone formation by stimulating osteoprogenitor cells to differentiate into osteoblasts. Osteoconduction is provided by biocompatible materials, which serve as a framework for bone growth in contact with their surface (ALBREKTSSON; JOHANSSON, 2001).

Although autogenous bone grafts are generally recognized as the gold standard for alveolar reconstruction, intraoral bone harvesting has been associated with an unsatisfactory amount of bone tissue and unpredictable graft resorption in the long term. In addition, the crestal incision used to gain access to the atrophic crest for bone insertion is associated with a high risk of dehiscence during the healing process, with exposure and consequent contamination and partial or total loss of the bone graft, thus compromising the final result of the reconstruction (RESTOY-LOZANO et al., 2015).

The healing of a bone graft is a dynamic process that includes the migration of mesenchymal cells from the surrounding bone marrow and differentiation into osteoblasts (OZKAN et al., 2007). Structurally, the ideal graft should have a thin layer of cortical bone and a predominance of medullary bone in order to simultaneously promote vascularization and nutrition as well as graft stability. In addition, proper immobilization of the graft is important to avoid micromovement and the consequent rupture of the newly formed vessels, which can lead to failure of the graft's incorporation into the recipient bed (RESTOY- LOZANO et al., 2015).

Buser et al. (1996) evaluated lateral bone crest augmentation with autogenous bone and a non-resorbable membrane. The clinical study involved 40 partially edentulous patients, only two of whom had unsatisfactory results. None of the bone blocks showed any clinical signs of resorption. The combination of membrane and autogenous bone is a predictable procedure for alveolar ridge augmentation. The bone graft supports the membrane and activates bone formation through its osteoconductive and osteoinductive properties.

Antoun et al. (2000) evaluated the use of two techniques for alveolar ridge augmentation using block autogenous bone alone or associated with the use of a non-absorbable membrane. Implants were successfully placed in all grafted sites. The average graft thickness was 4.7 mm (range: 2.3-6.2 mm). The average resorption was 1.5 mm (range: 0-4.6 mm), while the increase in width was 3.2 mm (range: 0.8-6.2 mm). Six months after surgery, the membrane group showed significantly less resorption than the non-membrane group. The increase in ridge width did not differ significantly between the two groups. In conclusion, the combination of a membrane with an autogenous block graft shows less bone resorption with a minimal risk of complications.

von Arx and Buser (2005) analyzed the clinical results of alveolar ridge augmentation using autogenous bone with inorganic bovine bone. A stepwise approach was used in 42 patients with severe horizontal bone atrophy. First, a bone graft was obtained from the mandibular symphysis or retromolar area and fixed with screws. The bone block was covered with inorganic bovine bone and a collagen membrane. After a period of six months, the implants were installed. Fifty-eight sites were regenerated, 41 of which were in the anterior maxillary region. The average initial ridge width was 3.06 mm and 7.66 mm after grafting. In conclusion, the authors demonstrated that the technique presented was successful in augmenting the alveolar ridge.

Elian et al. (2007) developed a classification of alveoli in which risks can be assessed in relation to the potential for recession depending on the existing condition. Type I alveoli are classified as having the buccal bone plate and soft tissue completely intact. Type II alveoli have the soft tissue present but there is a bone defect, indicating partial or complete lack of the buccal bone plate and type III alveoli indicate loss of the buccal bone and bone tissue.

Buser et al. (2008) in a case report discussed the advantages of early implant installation in an esthetic area. A 23-year-old female patient was referred to the clinic for extraction of her upper left central incisor due to complications arising from dental trauma. The surgical technique presented is characterized by the extraction of the tooth, without flap elevation, a soft tissue healing period of 4 to 8 weeks, placement of the implant in a correct three-dimensional position, augmentation of the ridge simultaneously on the buccal surface with guided bone regeneration using a resorbable collagen membrane combined with autogenous bone chips and a filling of bovine lyophilized bone and tension-free primary wound closure. The aim of this technique is to obtain a vestibular wall at least 3 mm thick. The use of a non-resorbable membrane is facilitated during surgery due to its hydrophilic characteristics. The most significant clinical advantage is that collagen membranes do not require a second surgical procedure to remove the membrane, as opposed to non-resorbable membranes. The aesthetic treatment in this case report, based on the concept of early implant installation, brings pleasing treatment results. In addition, the protocol is patient-friendly, as only one tissue detachment procedure is used and the time period from extraction to restoration with the provisional crown was around 16 weeks. However, a case report cannot be used to draw conclusions about the predictability of the concept presented; it can only present the clinical procedures and their biological basis.

Kumar et al. (2013) in a case report, described the use of a graft from the symphysis of the jaw for immediate implantation in an esthetic area. In the report, the patient treated had a fractured left upper central incisor. After extracting the fractured element, the implant was installed; however, a small space was present on the proximal and palatal surfaces of the implant, so it was decided to use autogenous bone to fill the spaces. The graft was obtained from the symphysis. A small incision was made in the apical region of the lower incisors to gain access to the bone tissue, from which a cylinder of bone tissue 11mm in diameter was removed using a trephine. The block was then broken into smaller pieces for insertion into the gap, covered with a resorbable membrane and sutured. A temporary crown was made to protect the recipient site. After six months, the definitive crown was made. The authors report that the symphysis region was chosen over the tuberosity due to the greater amount of bone tissue available. In conclusion, the authors recommend more cases with pre- and post-operative control.

Pierri et al. (2013) evaluated the aesthetic results and tissue stability of individual implants in the anterior maxillary region followed by reconstruction with autogenous mandibular bone covered with bovine hydroxyapatite and a resorbable collagen membrane over a five-year period. The patients selected were those with bone deficiency greater than or equal to three millimeters in the vertical and horizontal directions. The implants were installed six months after the regeneration procedures. The dimensions of the alveolar ridge were measured using computerized tomography. Clinical and radiographic measurements were taken annually to obtain the aesthetic parameters of the gingival tissue (pink aesthetic score - PES). The average bone gain was 4.23 ± 0.69 mm horizontally and 1.71 ± 0.75 mm vertically. The implant success rate was 100%. The average crestal bone resorption after 5 years was low (0.61 ± 0.33 mm). Moderate recession of the buccal mucosa (-1.12 ± 0.4 mm) was observed during the study period, while mesial and distal papilla heights increased slightly (0.13 ± 0.17 and 0.19 ± 0.37 mm, respectively). The mean PES remained stable, varying from 9.07 ± 1.49 at the time of permanent crown installation to 8.61 ± 1.55 in 5 years. Only two cases (7%) were considered slightly below the defined threshold (PES = 8) for marginal esthetic acceptability. In conclusion, the authors have shown that implants placed in maxillae that have received en bloc bone grafting have stable tissue levels and reasonable aesthetic results in the medium term.

In a clinical case study, Buser et al. (2013) evaluated 20 patients with implant-supported single crowns installed simultaneously with guided bone regeneration and followed up for 6 years. Clinical, radiographic and esthetic parameters were evaluated. In addition, computed tomography was used after 6 years to examine the thickness of the buccal bone wall. During the study period, all 20 implants were successfully integrated, and the clinical parameters remained stable over time. None of the implants showed mucosal recession of 1 mm or more. Periapical radiographs showed stable peri-implant bone levels. CT scans showed that all 20 implants had a detectable buccal bone wall at 6 years, with an average thickness of around 1.9 mm. The six-year follow-up showed that the risk of mucosal recession is low with early implant placement. In addition, contour augmentation with guided bone regeneration (GBR) was able to establish and maintain the buccal bone wall in all 20 patients.

According to Albrektsson and Isidor (1993) the success of an implant is shown when the bone margin loss is less than 1.5mm in the first year of function and less than 0.2mm in the following years. In 1999, Wennstrom and Palmer suggested modifying these criteria to a loss of no more than 2mm after a period of five years in function.

The areas commonly used as extra-oral donors are the iliac crest or tibia and the intra-oral areas are the mandibular symphysis and tuberosity (LIU; KERNS, 2014). Montazen et al. (2000) evaluated the amount of grafting material present in the mandibular symphysis, as well as determining the maximum zone for the collection of the coccygeal block, thus preventing damage to the teeth and other structures. Sixteen mandibles from dentate cadavers were studied. The osteotomy to remove the graft was performed monocortically, 5 mm in front of the mental foramen. The size of the bone block was measured using the volumetric displacement technique. The average graft size obtained was 4.84 ml. In conclusion, the authors demonstrate that the mandibular symphysis can be used as a site for bone graft collection. Hassani et al. (2005) evaluated the amount of bone graft that could be obtained from the anterior region of the palate in a cadaver study. Twenty-one cadavers, both dentate and edentulous, were studied. The osteotomy was performed monocortically, 2 mm from the alveolar bone crest and parallel to the tooth axis and 3 mm from the incisive foramen in the midline. Drill penetration was indicated by a radiographic index. The amount of corticospongy block was then measured using the volumetric displacement technique. The average bone volume obtained was 2.03 ml in toothed cadavers and 2.40 ml in edentulous cadavers. Based on the results of this study, the anterior region of the palate can be reliably used as a donor site in reconstructive surgery, implantology and periodontal regeneration procedures.

Although the use of autogenous bone grafts covered by membranes is considered the gold standard for effective bone regeneration, due to their biocompatibility and faster regeneration of lost hard tissue, some studies and clinical case reports have shown that comparable results can be obtained when using non-autogenous graft materials covered by a suitable membrane (DINATO et al. 2007).

Xenogeneic bone

Xenografts, or xenograft bone substitutes, consist of animal-derived bone mineral or bone-like materials derived from calcified coral or algae, from which the organic component is removed to eliminate the risk of immunogenic response or disease transmission (BUSER, 2010).

Xenografts derived from natural bone sources have been extensively researched in various clinical and experimental studies. In particular, medullary bovine bone has been used as a source of these substitutes due to its proximity to human medullary bone. The organic component is removed by heat treatment, chemical extraction method or a combination of both to eliminate the risk of immune responses and disease transmission (BUSER, 2010).

Bone grafts can be classified in relation to the biological properties they have when installed in the recipient bed. These properties are osteoconduction, osteinduction and osteogenesis (DINOPOULOS, 2012). Osteoconduction is the ability of the graft to aid healing through its micro and macroscopic framework, allowing vascular infiltration and the internal migration of cellular elements involved in bone formation such as undifferentiated mesenchymal cells, osteoblasts, osteoclasts, among others. Normally, osteoconduction is more efficient when other properties such as osteinduction and osteogenesis are present in the same material. Osteoconduction seems to be optimized in devices that mimic not only the physical structure of bone, but also its chemical composition (GIANNOUDIS, 2005). Two important conditions must be met for successful osteoconduction: (1) the framework must consist of a bioactive material or bioinert, and (2) the shape and dimensions of its internal and external structures must favor invagination and bone deposition (BUSER, 2010).

Salama (1983), in a clinical study, used bone of xenogenic origin mixed with bone marrow from 98 patients. The results were satisfactory, suggesting that xenogenic bone has a wide range of uses.

Nyman et al. (1990) in a report of two clinical cases, used the principle of guided tissue regeneration to regenerate alveolar bone tissue concomitantly with the installation of implants. In one case, implant osseointegration was achieved by placing a Teflon membrane along the implant inserted into a post-extraction socket. In a second case, the same biological principle was used to increase the bone volume of an alveolar ridge without teeth to provide the appropriate dimensions for implant installation. In both cases, the membrane seems to have prevented the repopulation of the wound area by connective tissue cells, allowing only bone-derived cells to repopulate in the space between the membrane.

Hammerle et al. (1998) in an in vivo study, tested the effect of deproteinized bovine bone used for guided bone regeneration in defects around implants. All 2 first molars and premolars were extracted from both sides of the mandibles of 3 monkeys (Macaca fascicularis). After three months, two implants were installed in all quadrants of each monkey. During the surgical procedure, standardized defects were produced in the buccal and lingual bone wall, measuring 2.5 mm in width and 3 mm in height. Four different experimental situations were created: two sites in each monkey were covered with an ePTFE membrane (M), two sites were filled with the grafting material (DBBM), two sites were filled with the grafting material and also covered with a membrane (M + DBBM), and two sites were neither grafted nor covered with a membrane, serving as a control (C). Linear measurements of bone height and width were calculated on histological specimens obtained 6 months after surgery. Vertical bone growth along the implant surface was 100% (SD 0%) for M + DBBM, 91% (SD 9%) for M, 52% (SD 24%) for DBBM, and 42% (SD 35%) for C. The width of the regenerated bone amounted to 97% (SD 2%) for M + DBBM, 85% (SD 9%) for M, 42% (SD 41%) for DBBM, and 23% (SD 31%) for C. In conclusion, deproteinized bovine bone (Bio-Oss) exhibited osteoconductive properties and can therefore be recommended for GBR procedures in bone defects, both horizontally and vertically.

Hammerle and Lang (2001) evaluated in a clinical trial whether peri-implant bone defects can be regenerated with deproteinized bovine bone and resorbable membranes simultaneously with implant installation. Three women and seven men aged between 32 and 68 years (average 54.5) were included in the study. Eight to 14 weeks after atraumatic tooth extraction, the implants were placed in the extraction sites. At this point, all the implants had alveolar bone defects, partly exposing the implant threads. Guided bone regeneration was carried out using deproteinized bovine bone (BioOss) and bioabsorbable collagen membrane (Bio-Gide) as a barrier. Clinical measurements were taken at 6 sites around each implant (mid-vestibular, vestibular, disto-vestibular, disto-lingual, lingual, mesio-lingual), using a calibrated periodontal probe. At the beginning of the study, the average defect depth per patient was 3.6 mm (standard deviation 1.6 mm, range 1.8-6.8 mm). The deepest defects were located on the buccal surfaces (mean 7.8 millimeters, SD 1.9 mm). On re-entry, the depth had decreased to 2.5 mm (SD 0.6 millimeters). This difference was statistically significant (P<0.01). Initially, in 62% of the sites the depth ranged from 0-3 mm, in 23% it ranged from 2-4 mm, and in 15% to more than 6 mm. Six to seven months later, at re-entry, 95% of sites were less than 3 mm and 5% depth and ranged from 4-6 mm. Defect coverage, as assessed by the amount of implant surface exposed, reached an average value of 86% (SD 33%). In eight implants there was total coverage (100%), 60% in one and 0% in another implant, which showed signs of infection during healing. Thus, the authors concluded that resorbable materials in GBR procedures simultaneously with implant installation can lead to bone regeneration in peri-implant defects.

Norton et al. (2003) in a study to evaluate the osteoconductivity of bovine mineral bone in humans, evaluated fifteen patients treated for the repair of alveolar defects and/or ridge maintenance after exodontia, prior to the installation of implants. Bovine mineral bone was used as the main grafting material to fill the sites. Bone cylinders were removed to evaluate the tissue response under the microscope. A total of 22 cylinders were obtained for histomorphometric evaluation to calculate the average percentage of bone, residual graft and connective tissue. In addition, the average percentage of bone-graft contact was also calculated. The average percentage of new bone formation was 26.9%, and the percentage of residual graft and connective tissue was 25.6% and 47.4%, respectively. The average contact between bone and residual graft was 34%. One implant installed in a site that was histologically identified as having little new bone and, exceptionally, an inflammatory infiltrate, failed, showing mobility. All the other implants were restored to function, with a baseline survival rate of 97%. The authors concluded that bovine mineral bone demonstrated osteoconductive capacity for the formation of new bone.

De Boever and De Boever (2003) described cases of fenestration in narrow ridges at the time of implant installation. The exposed parts of the implants were covered with deproteinized bovine bone (Bio-Oss) and a non-resorbable PTFE-e membrane. The fenestrations ranged from 5 to 8.5 mm. The membranes were removed after 12 to 20 weeks. One of the seven implants failed to osseointegrate. In four cases, there was no residual defect (100% coverage). In two cases, 63.5% and 87.5% coverage was achieved, respectively. During follow-up from one year and five months to four years and seven months after implant installation, the clinical probing depth never exceeded 3.5 mm. Radiographically, no resorption was found. The authors' conclusion was that, in selected cases, fenestrae can be successfully treated using deproteinized bovine bone in combination with non-resorbable membranes.

Meijndert et al. (2005) investigated the quality of the bone tissue formed in areas grafted in the anterior maxillary region. Reconstruction was carried out using autogenous bone, autogenous bone and resorbable membrane and deproteinized bovine bone (Bio-Oss) and membrane. In the areas where only autogenous bone was used, sites with non-vital bone and sites with bone apposition and remodeling were observed. Similar results were observed in the sites reconstructed with autogenous graft covered with membrane. In the group that used Bio-Oss, newly formed bone tissue was observed around the particle of material, but most of the particles were surrounded by connective tissue. At the time of implant placement, the grafting material was still present and had not been completely replaced by vital bone. Despite the differences, after one year of clinical follow-up the results were satisfactory when comparing the grafting techniques.

Juodzbalys and Wang (2007) in a case series clinically and radiographically evaluated the esthetic results of implants installed in fresh alveoli. Twelve patients received 14 implants, ranging from 13 to 16 mm in size and 4.3 to 5 mm in diameter. The defects after implant installation were measured and then filled with deproteinized bovine bone with a resorbable membrane. The defect was re-evaluated at reopening. The clinical and radiographic parameters of the peri-implant conditions were established at the time of prosthesis installation and followed up for one year. The implant success rate was 100% after one year. Analysis of the esthetic results showed that the average "pink esthetic" score was 11.1 (SD 1.35) at one-year follow-up. During the follow-up period, the distance between the implant shoulder and the bone crest remained stable. Careful assessment before extraction and implant installation promotes an optimal aesthetic result. Sites with compromised bone volume can be successfully corrected using guided bone regeneration.

Hammerle et al. (2008) tested whether the use of resorbable membranes and xenogenous bone substitutes allows horizontal augmentation of the ridge in place of autogenous grafting, allowing the installation of implants under normal conditions. Twelve patients in need of implants took part in the study. The flaps were carefully detached and blocks or particles of deproteinized bovine bone (DBBM) (Bio-Oss) were placed in the defect area. A collagen membrane (Bio-Gide) was used to cover the DBBM and fixed to the surrounding bone using poly-L-lactic acid pins. The flaps were sutured to allow healing by first intention. No dehiscence or membrane exposure was observed. Nine to 10 months after the augmentation surgery, the flaps were lifted in order to visualize the results of the augmentation. An integration of the DBBM particles into the newly formed bone was consistently observed. In all but one case, the bone volume after regeneration was suitable for installing the implants in an ideal position.

Before the regenerative procedure, the average width of the bone crest was 3.2 mm and 6.9 mm at the time of implant placement. This difference was statistically significant. After a healing period of 9-10 months, the combination of DBBM and collagen membrane proved to be an effective treatment option for horizontal bone augmentation prior to implant placement.

Myamoto and Obama (2011) evaluated the influence of labial alveolar bone thickness and corresponding vertical bone loss on post-operative gingival recessions around implants in the anterior maxilla. Using single-beam computed tomography, the changes in the three-dimensional images of the alveolar bone were monitored to determine the results for the hard and soft tissue of two implant installation techniques: two-stage and immediate. In addition, for two-stage installation, guided bone regeneration was adopted, using non-resorbable or resorbable membranes combined with inorganic bovine bone matrix. The comparative results suggested that gingival recessions were significantly lower in two-stage placement, especially when using a non-resorbable membrane, compared to immediate installation. The thickness of the buccal bone, measured by CBCT, provided an effective indicator for assessing gingival recession in the anterior region.

In a case series, Grunder, Wenz and Schupbach (2011) evaluated the clinical and histological results of GBR on simultaneously installed implants. To be included in the study, patients had to have a defect in the buccal bone wall. Eight patients were included in the study, with an average defect of 4 mm. After implant installation, the defects were filled with mineralized bovine bone (Bio-Oss) and a non-resorbable membrane. After six months, the membrane was removed and the site biopsied for histological assessment. The clinical results showed adequate tissue volume. No implants were lost during the evaluation period. The histological sections showed various amounts of new bone, bovine bone particles and medullary space. The formation of bone tissue was evident in the presence of osteoid matrix and osteoblasts. The authors concluded that the method presented is clinically controllable and that it is possible to obtain good aesthetic results in the anterior maxilla, with a good prognosis and longevity. In the histological evaluation, the authors demonstrated that bone formation occurred.

Furze et al. (2011) evaluated the clinical and esthetic results of 10 cases with single implants in esthetic areas. The treatment protocol consisted of: (1) atraumatic extraction; (2) installation of the implant simultaneously with guided bone regeneration (Bio-Oss and Bio-Guide) 6-8 weeks after extraction; (3) installation of the provisional 2 to 3 months after implant installation; (4) molding; (5) installation of the abutment and definitive crown six months after installation of the provisional. The results were measured one year after the installation of the definitive crown. All implants had 100% survival. According to the authors, the use of the treatment protocol described can promote an aesthetically pleasing treatment for single implants in the anterior maxillary region.

Block, Ducote and Mercante (2012) evaluated the stability of particulate xenografts and membranes in the anterior maxilla. The authors hypothesized that particulate material under a collagen membrane would be a reliable and predictable bone augmentation method for use in the maxilla. Twelve patients received bovine particulate grafts and were evaluated retrospectively. Using a standardized method, cone beam CT scans were obtained and measured at 3 vertical locations preoperatively (T0), immediately after augmentation (T1), 3 to 6 months after augmentation and before implant placement (T2), immediately after implant placement (T3) and at the longest point postoperatively (T4). An examiner, who was not involved in the surgical procedures, measured all the CT scans. As a result, the most coronal part of the ridge had a smaller increase in width. The central region and the apical region had the greatest changes (P <.001). Within the sample size, there were no statistically significant differences in the changes in width over time after the augmentation was performed. Within the limitations of this sample, horizontal ridge augmentation using bovine particulate material under a membrane proves to be stable over time, being a simpler method to perform and with less morbidity for the patient, being considered an alternative to autogenous grafting.

Buser et al. (2013) in a prospective cross-sectional study, evaluated 41 patients with a single implant in an esthetic region on two occasions (2006 and 2010) using clinical, radiographic and esthetic parameters. All the patients showed stability, with no signs of peri-implantitis. The clinical parameters remained stable over time and the aesthetic results were satisfactory. None of the implants showed mucosal recession over time, as confirmed by the distance between the implant shoulder and the mucosal margin. Periapical radiographs showed stable peri-implant bone levels, with an average distance between the implant shoulder and the implant thread of 2.18 mm. CBCT analysis showed an average thickness of the buccal bone wall of 2.2 mm. In two implants (4.9%) no facial bone wall was detected by radiography. The conclusions of this study demonstrate the stability of the hard and soft tissue around the implant and satisfactory esthetics. The 5 to 9-year follow-up confirmed that the risk of gingival recession is low with early implant installation. In addition, GBR was able to establish and maintain buccal bone in 95% of patients.

Suleimenova et al. (2016) studied the expression of genes related to guided bone regeneration in the initial phase of the process, combined with different biomaterials. Skull defects in four New Zealand rabbits were filled with A) experimental pericardium-derived collagen membrane, B) Bio-Oss/Bio-Gide, C) bifacial calcium phosphate/hydroxyapatite-containing collagen membrane and D) Bio-Oss/hydroxyapatite-containing collagen membrane. Seven days after surgery, one animal was assessed histologically and the other three were subjected to real-time PCR (qPCR). The analysis showed that 9 of the 84 genes in the sequence were significantly different in the three experimental groups (groups A, C and D). Group D showed the greatest change in gene expression after seven days. The genes that had significantly decreased expression (AHSG, EGF) or increased expression (CDH11, MMP13, GLI1 and MCSF) are responsible for the initial stage of bone formation, bone remodeling and pre-osteoclast development. The patterns of gene expression in the initial healing phase of defects treated with GBR appear to be related to the biomaterial used. The combination of Bio-Oss and collagen membrane containing hydroxyapatite showed the most pro-osteogenic gene regulation profile (group D), which implies the stimulation of important transcription factors, which implies earlier bone formation.

MATERIALS AND METHODS

This literature review included a search for scientific articles indexed in the Pubmed database, using the following keywords: Esthetics, Guided bone regeneration (GBR), Dental Implant, Long-term, Follow-up.

We also consulted articles in Portuguese from the Internet, book chapters and monographs, dissertations and theses from the main centers of specialization in the country.

DISCUSSION

Guided bone regeneration is a bone reconstruction technique that uses membranes to promote the growth and development of bone tissue, which grows more slowly than other tissues. The membrane acts as a barrier, creating a space for osteoprogenitor cells and the formation of blood vessels, which carry oxygen and undifferentiated mesenchymal cells to the grafted site.

The bone substitutes used in this study were autogenous bone and xenogeneic bone. The purpose of these materials is to support the membrane and prevent it from collapsing; to serve as a framework for bone invagination from the recipient bed; to stimulate bone invagination from the recipient bed; to provide a mechanical barrier against pressure from the overlying soft tissue and; to protect the increased volume from being resorbed (BUSER, 2010).

Autogenous bone has been chosen as the main material for en bloc bone reconstruction, as it is the only one with the three fundamental characteristics for bone repair and graft maintenance: osteoconduction, osteoinduction and osteogenesis, the latter being exclusive to this material. However, the use of autogenous bone has some disadvantages. It is a second surgical site and its removal increases post-operative morbidity. Due to the limited amount of bone in intraoral donor sites, an extraoral approach may be necessary for certain reconstructions (NYSTROM et al., 2009; ROTHAMEL et al., 2009).

Xenografts derived from natural bone sources have been extensively researched in various clinical and experimental studies. In particular, medullary bovine bone has been used as a source of these substitutes due to its proximity to human medullary bone (BUSER, 2010). Of the three fundamental biological properties, xenogeneic bone only possesses osteconduction. This characteristic allows the cells that enabled bone neofromation to grow. For successful osteoconduction, the material must meet two conditions: it must be a bioactive or bioinert framework and it must be similar in shape and size to natural bone. The large internal surface area similar to human bone facilitates the absorption of endogenous proteins and growth factors, as does the chemical composition analogous to human bone with few hydroxyls and more carbonate groupings than other synthetic materials. The size of the crystals, comparable to human bone, can facilitate their absorption, and their special natural porous architecture with a trabeculation very similar to human bone promotes better revascularization and also maintains a framework for osteoconductivity, increasing the stabilization of the hinge and natural blood absorption between the micros and macropores (ARTZI, TAL, DAYAN 2000).

Pierri et al. (2013) and Buser et al. (2013) reported high implant survival rates in sites that showed guided bone regeneration using autogenous grafts. In addition, the esthetic parameters remained stable during the evaluation period.

Grunder, Wenz and Schupbach (2011) and Block, Ducote and Mercante (2012) also demonstrated high success rates in cases using xenogeneic grafts, considering this type of material an alternative to autogenous grafts.

CONCLUSION

Based on the above, we conclude:

- Guided bone regeneration is a predictable, long-term stable procedure;

- Autogenous and xenogenous materials demonstrate longevity in treatment;

- Autogenous grafts are used for larger reconstructions, such as horizontal and vertical augmentations, and xenogeneic grafts for smaller fillings, such as fenestrations.

REFERENCES

WENNERBERG, A, ALBREKTSSON, T. Current challenges in successful rehabilitation with oral implants. *Journal of Oral Rehabilitation*. v. 38, n. 4, p. 286-294, 2011.

SHARMA, P. et. al. Implant esthetic restoration in ridge deficiencies in cases of trauma: a case report. *Journal of Oral Rehabilitation*. DOI: 10.1563/AAID-JOI-D-I 100181

AMOROSO, A. P. et. al. Reverse planning in implant dentistry: clinical case report. *Revista Odontológica de Araçatuba*. v. 33, n.2, p. 75-79. 2012.

ALOY-PRÓSPER A, PENARROCHA-OLTRA D, PENARROCHA-DIAGO MA, PENARROCHA-DIAGO M. The outcome of intraoral onlay block bone grafts on alveo- lar ridge augmentations: A systematic review. *Medicina Oral Patologia y Cirugia Bucal*. v. 20, n. 2, p. 251-258, 2015.

FARZAD, M., MOHAMMADI, M. Guided bone regeneration: A literature review. *Journal of Oral Health and Oral Epidemiology*. v. 1, n. 1, p. 3-18, 2012.

WANG H.L., CARROLL M.J. Guided bone regeneration using bone grafts and collagen membranes. *Quintessence International*. v. 32, p. 504-515, 2001.

CLEMENTINI, M., MORLUPI, A., CANULLO, L., AGRESTINI, C., BARLATTANI, A.

Success rate of dental implants inserted in horizontal and vertical guided bone regenerated areas: a systematic review. *International Journal of Oral & Maxillofacial Surgery*. v. 41, p. 847-852, 2012.

CLEMENTINI, M., MORLUPI, A., AGRESTINI, C., BARLATTANI, A. Immediate versus delayed positioning of dental implants in guided bone regeneration or onlay graft regenerated areas: a systematic review. *International Journal of Oral & Maxillofacial Surgery*. v. 42, p.643-650, 2013.

CHEN, S. T., BUSER, D. Clinical and esthetic outcomes of implants placed in postextraction sites. *International Journal of Oral & Maxillofacial Implants*. v. 24, p. 186-217, 2009.

BUSER, D., CHAPPUIS, V., KUCHLER, U., BORNSTEIN, M.M., WITTNEBEN, J.G., BUSER, R., CAVUSOGLU, Y., BELSER, U.C. Long-term stability of early implant placement with contour augmentation. *Journal of Dental Research*. v. 92, n. 12, p. 176-182, 2013.

DINATO, José Cicero ; NUNES, L. S. S. ; SMIDT, Ricardo . Surgical techniques for bone regeneration, enabling the installation of implants. In: Eduardo Saba-Chufji ; Silvio Antonio dos Santos Pereira. (Org.). Periodontology: Integration and results. Sâo Paulo. p. 183-226. 2007.

BUSER D, 20 Years of Guided Bone Regeneration in Implant Dentistry. São Paulo: Quintessence; 2010.

MCALLISTER B.S, HAGHIGHAT K. Bone augmentation techniques. *Journal of Periodontology. v. 78, n. 3, p. 377-396. 2007*

FURLANETO, F.A., NAGATA, M.J., FUCINI, S.E., DELIBERADOR, T.M., OKAMOTO, T., MESSORA, M.R. Bone healing in critical-size defects treated with bioactive glass/ calcium sulfate: a histologic and histometric study in rat calvaria. *Clinical Oral Implants Research*, v. 18, p. 311-318, 2007.

DELIBERADOR T, NAGATA M, FURLANETO F, MELO L, OKAMOTO T, SUNDEFELD M, ET AL. Autogenous bone graft with or without a calcium sulfate barrier in the treatment of Class II furcation defects: a histologic and histometric study in dogs. *Journal of Periodontology. v. 77, n. 5, p. 780-789. 2006.*

ALBREKTSSON T, JOHANSSON C. Osteoinduction, osteoconduction and osseointegration. *European Spine Journal.* v. 10, n. 2, p.96-101. 2001.

RESTOY-LOZANO, J.L. DOMINGUEZ-MOMPELL, P. INFANTE-COSSIO, J. LARA-CHAO, F. ESPIN-GALVEZ, V. LOPEZ-PIZARRO. Reconstruction of mandibular vertical defects for dental implants with autogenous bone block grafts using a tunnel approach: clinical study of 50 cases. *International Journal of Oral & Maxillofacial Surgery.* v. 44, n. 11, p. 1416-1422. 2015.

OZKAN Y, OZCAN M, VAROL A, AKOGLU B, UCANKALE M, BASA S. Resonance frequency analysis assessment of implant stability in labial onlay grafted posterior mandibles: a pilot clinical study. *International Journal of Oral & Maxillofacial Implants.* v. 22, n. 2, p 235-242. 2007.

BUSER R, DULA K, HIRT H.P, SCHENK, R. K. Lateral ridge augmentation using autografts and barrier membranes: A clinical study with 40 partially edentulous patients. *Journal of Oral and Maxillofacial Surgery.* v. 54, n. 4, p. 420-432. 1996.

ANTOUN H, SITBON JM, MARTINEZ H, MISSIKA P. A prospective randomized study comparing two techniques of bone augmentation: onlay graft alone or associated with a membrane. *Clinical Oral Implants Research*, v. 12, p. 632-639. 2007.

VON ARX T, BUSER D. Horizontal ridge augmentation using autogenous block grafts and the guided bone regeneration technique with collagen membranes: a clinical study with 42 patients. *Clinical Oral Implants Research. v.* 17, p. 359-366. 2006

ELIAN N, CHO S.C, FROUM S, SMITH R.B, TARNOW D.P. A simplified socket classification and repair technique. *Practical procedures & aesthetic dentistry.* v. 19, n. 2, p. 99-104. 2007.

BUSER D, CHEN S.T, WEBER H.P, BELSER U.C. Early implant placement following single-tooth extraction in the esthetic zone: biologic rationale and surgical procedures. *International Journal of Periodontics & Restorative Dentistry.* v. 28, n. 5, p. 441-451. 2008.

KUMAR N.S, SOWMYA N, MEHTA D.S, KUMAR P.S. Minimal guided bone regeneration procedure for immediate implant placement in the esthetic zone. *Dental Research Journal.* v. 10, n. 1, p. 98-102. 2013.

PIERI F, ALDINI N.N, MARCHETTI C, CORINALDESI G. Esthetic outcome and tissue stability of maxillary anterior single-tooth implants following reconstruction with mandibular block grafts: a 5-year prospective study. *International Journal of Oral & Maxillofacial Implants.* v. 28, n. 1, p. 270-280. 2013

BUSER D, CHAPPUIS V, KUCHLER U, BORNSTEIN M.M, WITTNEBEN J.G, BUSER R, CAVUSOGLU Y, BELSER U.C. Long-term stability of early implant placement with contour augmentation. *Journal of Dental Research.* v. 92, n. 12, p. 176-182. 2013.

Albrektsson T., Isidor F. (1993). Consensus report of session IV, in Proceedings of the 1st European Workshop on Periodontology, eds Lang N. P., Karring T., editors (London: Quintessence;), 365-369

Wennstrom J., Palmer R. (1999). Consensus report session 3: clinical trials, in Proceedings of the 3rd European Workshop on Periodontology. Implant Dentistry, eds Lang N. P., Karring T., Lindhe J., editors (Berlin: Quintessence;), 345-350

LIU J, KERNS D.G. Mechanisms of guided bone regeneration: a review. *Open Dentistry Journal.* v. 16, n. 8, p. 56-65. 2014

MONTAZEM A, VALAURI D.V, ST-HILAIRE H, BUCHBINDER D. The mandibular symphysis as a donor site in maxillofacial bone grafting: a quantitative anatomic study. *Journal of Oral and Maxillofacial Surgery.* v. 58, n. 12, p. 1368-1371. 2000.

HASSANI A, KHOJASTEH A, SHAMSABAD A.N. The anterior palate as a donor site in maxillofacial bone grafting: a quantitative anatomic study. *Journal of Oral and Maxillofacial*

Surgery. v. 63, n. 8, p. 1196-1200. 2005.

NANDI S.K, ROY S, MUKHERJEE P, KUNDU B, DE D.K, BASU D. Orthopaedic applications of bone graft & graft substitutes : a review. *Indian Journal of Medical Research.* v. 132, n. 1, p. 15-30. 2010.

Giannoudis P.V, Dinopoulos H, Tsiridis E. Bone substitutes: an update. *Injury.* v. 36, n. 3, p. 20-27. 2005.

SALAMA, R. Xenogeneic bone grafting in humans. *Clinical orthopaedics and related research,* v. 174, p. 113-121, 1983.

NYMAN, S et al. Bone regeneration adjacent to titanium dental implants using guided tissue regeneration: a report of two cases. *International Journal of Oral & Maxillofacial Implants,* v. 5, n. 1, 1990.

HAMMERLE, C.H.F et al. The effect of a deproteinized bovine bone mineral on bone regeneration around titanium dental implants. *Clinical Oral Implants Research.* v. 9, n. 3, p. 151-162, 1998.

HAMMERLE, C.H.F; LANG, N. P. Single stage surgery combining transmucosal implant placement with guided bone regeneration and bioresorbable materials. *Clinical Oral Implants Research,* v. 12, n. 1, p. 9-18, 2001.

NORTON, M.R. et al. Efficacy of bovine bone mineral for alveolar augmentation: a human histologic study. *Clinical Oral Implants Research,* v. 14, n. 6, p. 775-783, 2003.

DE BOEVER, L, DE BOEVER, J. A. A one-stage approach for nonsubmerged implants using a xenograft in narrow ridges: report on seven cases. *International Journal of Periodontics & Restorative Dentistry,* v. 23, n. 2, 2003.

MEIJNDERT, L. et al. Bone quality at the implant site after reconstruction of a local defect of the maxillary anterior ridge with chin bone or deproteinized cancellous bovine bone. *International journal of oral and maxillofacial surgery,* v. 34, n. 8, p. 877884, 2005.

JUODZBALYS, G; WANG, H. Soft and hard tissue assessment of immediate implant placement: a case series. *Clinical Oral Implants Research,* v. 18, n. 2, p. 237-243, 2007.

HAMMERLE, C.H.F et al. Ridge augmentation by applying bioresorbable membranes and deproteinized bovine bone mineral: a report of twelve consecutive cases. *Clinical oral implants research,* v. 19, n. 1, p. 19-25, 2008.

MIYAMOTO, Y; OBAMA, T. Dental cone beam computed tomography analyses of postoperative labial bone thickness in maxillary anterior implants: comparing immediate and delayed implant placement. *International Journal of Periodontics and Restorative Dentistry*, v. 31, n. 3, p. 215, 2011.

GRUNDER, U; WENZ, B; SCHUPBACH, P. Guided bone regeneration around single-tooth implants in the esthetic zone: a case series. *International Journal of Periodontics and Restorative Dentistry*, v. 31, n. 6, p. 613, 2011.

FURZE, D et al. Clinical and esthetic outcomes of single-tooth implants in the anterior maxilla. *Quintessence International*, v. 43, n. 2, 2012.

BLOCK, M.S.; DUCOTE, C. W.; MERCANTE, D. E. Horizontal augmentation of thin maxillary ridge with bovine particulate xenograft is stable during 500 days of followup: preliminary results of 12 consecutive patients. *Journal of Oral and Maxillofacial Surgery,* v. 70, n. 6, p. 1321-1330, 2012.

BUSER, D. et al. Long-term stability of contour augmentation with early implant placement following single tooth extraction in the esthetic zone: a prospective, cross-sectional study in 41 patients with a 5-to 9-year follow-up. *Journal of periodontology*, v. 84, n. 11, p. 1517-1527, 2013.

SULEIMENOVA, D. et al. Gene expression profiles in guided bone regeneration using combinations of different biomaterials: a pilot animal study. *Clinical oral implants research*, 2016.

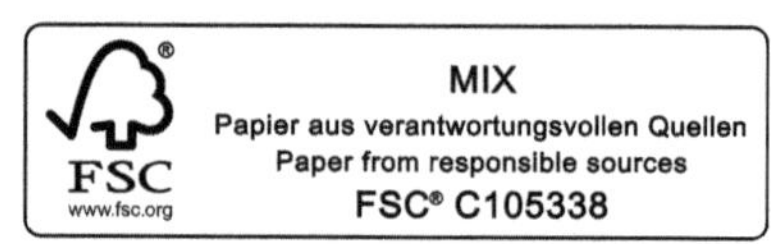

Printed by Books on Demand GmbH, Norderstedt / Germany